A Statistical Inqui[ry]

Nature and Treatme[nt]

Alexander Hughes Bennett

Alpha Editions

This edition published in 2024

ISBN : 9789362097217

Design and Setting By
Alpha Editions
www.alphaedis.com
Email - info@alphaedis.com

As per information held with us this book is in Public Domain.
This book is a reproduction of an important historical work. Alpha Editions uses the best technology to reproduce historical work in the same manner it was first published to preserve its original nature. Any marks or number seen are left intentionally to preserve its true form.

I.

AN ENQUIRY INTO THE ETIOLOGY AND SYMPTOMATOLOGY OF EPILEPSY.[A]

The science of medicine is to be advanced by the careful collection of well-recorded facts, rather than by general statements or unsupported assertions. No inquiry thus conducted with scientific precision can fail to be without value, and to add a mite to that store of positive knowledge from which must emanate all hopes of progress for the healing art. Our acquaintance with the nature of epilepsy is as yet in its infancy, and although much valuable practical information has been put on record regarding this disease, it is believed that the following contribution may not be useless in either confirming or questioning previous conclusions.

The clinical aspects of epilepsy are especially difficult to investigate with exactitude. The physician, as a rule, is not himself a witness to the chief phenomena characteristic of the disease. He is therefore compelled, in most cases, to trust to the statements of the patient and his friends for their description, and even when the cross-examination is conducted with the greatest care, there are many points impossible to ascertain with certainty. In the following cases of epilepsy, which have been under my own care, those only are included in which loss of consciousness formed the chief feature of the attack; and in the succeeding particulars, attention will be specially directed to etiology and symptomatology.

ETIOLOGY.

This may conveniently be discussed under (1) Predisposing causes, and (2) Exciting causes.

1.—PREDISPOSING CAUSES.

Sex and Sexual Conditions.—In one hundred unselected cases of epilepsy there were—

                Males,   47 per cent.

Females, 53 per cent.

showing that practically the sexes were affected in equal proportions. Of the females there were—

Unmarried, 58.5 per cent.

Married, 41.5 per cent.

The greater number amongst the unmarried females is probably due to the list including children, and also to the fact that epilepsy is not an attraction to a man who purposes matrimony. Of the married females—

The attacks were uninfluenced by marriage in 68.1 per cent.

The attacks were diminished after marriage in 27.2 per cent.

The attacks were increased after marriage in 4.5 per cent.

Thus, in the majority of cases, marriage seems to have no influence on the epileptic attacks of women, although in 27.2 per cent. the fits appear to have been diminished after that ceremony.

Of the married females there were—

Children in 82.3 per cent.

No children in 17.6 per cent.

Age.—In one hundred cases the age at which the first attack of epilepsy took place will be seen from the following tables:—

	Males.	Females.	Total.
From 1 to 10 years	9	14	23
From 10 to 20 years	11	23	34
From 20 to 30 years	14	9	23
From 30 to 40 years	10	6	16
From 40 to 50 years	1	0	1
From 50 to 60 years	2	1	3

It will thus be seen that, in males, the most prevalent period for the first invasion of epilepsy is from the tenth to the thirtieth year; in females, from the first to the twentieth year. In both sexes the disease rarely commences after forty. The following table shows the ages of the patients under observation:—

	Males.	Females.	Total.
From 1 to 10 years	4	1	5
From 0 to 20 years	10	20	30
From 20 to 30 years	17	15	32
From 30 to 40 years	11	9	20
From 40 to 50 years	2	6	8
From 50 to 60 years	3	2	5

This indicates that cases of epilepsy comparatively rarely come under observation after the age of forty. A large series of cases would however be required to determine any definite conclusions as to the mortality and longevity of the patients.

Occupation and Profession.—These do not appear to have any special relation to the production of epilepsy.

Hereditary Tendency.—In each of the cases under observation a very careful inquiry was made into the family history. This was confined to the parents, grand parents, uncles, aunts, brothers, sisters, and children of the patient. The following are the results:—

No family history of epilepsy, insanity, nervous or other hereditary disorders in 59 per cent.

One or more members of family affected with one or more of the above disorders in 41 per cent.

Of these last, in which there was a tainted hereditary history, one or more members of the family suffered from—

Epilepsy in	63.4 per cent.
Insanity in	12.1 per cent.
Phthisis in	12.1 per cent.
Asthma in	2.4 per cent.
Apoplexy in	2.4 per cent.
Hysteria in	2.4 per cent.
Hemiplegia in	2.4 per cent.
Spinal complaint in	2.4 per cent.

Concerning the above table, it is to be remarked that frequently the patient had several relatives suffering from different diseases; for example, one with epilepsy, a second with insanity, and so on. In such a case these have been classified under epilepsy, and, if this did not exist, under insanity, or other afflictions in the above order.

Of those cases in which epilepsy was present in the family of the patient, it existed in the following members:—

Father in	11.5 per cent.
Mother in	7.6 per cent.
Father, mother, and brother in	3.8 per cent.
Mother and child in	3.8 per cent.
Grandmother, mother, and two sisters in	3.8 per cent.
Mother and sister in	3.8 per cent.
Grandfather in	7.6 per cent.
Grandmother in	3.8 per cent.
Brother in	11.5 per cent.
Sister in	11.5 per cent.
Two brothers in	3.8 per cent.
Sister and child in	7.6 per cent.
Brother and uncle in	3.8 per cent.
Two uncles in	3.8 per cent.
Uncle in	3.8 per cent.
Aunt in	3.8 per cent.
Child in	3.8 per cent.

From these figures it will be seen that in no less than 41 per cent. of the total number of cases there was a distinct family history of hereditary disease. Of these no less than 87.5 per cent. were affections of the nervous system, and 12.1 per cent. of phthisis. Of the former 63.4 per cent. had relatives afflicted with epilepsy, and 12.1 per cent. with insanity. Epilepsy, according to these figures is eminently a hereditary disease, and it is possible even to a greater extent than is here represented; for the family history is often very difficult to arrive at, in the class of persons on whom most of these observations were made, who, either from ignorance or from prejudice, display a great want of knowledge concerning the health of their ancestors.

General health prior to the first attack.—As far as could be ascertained this was—

>Unimpaired in 90 per cent.
>
>Delicate in 10 per cent.

By the term delicate is understood any chronic derangement of health. The figures serve to indicate that, in the large majority of cases epilepsy has no necessary connection with the impaired general health of the patient.

Special illnesses prior to the first attack.—There were—

>No antecedent diseases in 78 per cent.
>
>Antecedent diseases in 32 per cent.

Of these persons who, prior to the first attack of epilepsy, had suffered from illnesses, the details are as follows:—

>Convulsions at dentition in 43.7 per cent.
>
>Rheumatic fever in 12.5 per cent.
>
>Chorea in 6.2 per cent.
>
>Mental derangement in 6.2 per cent.
>
>Constant headache in 6.2 per cent.
>
>Suppurating glands in 3.1 per cent.
>
>Brain fever (?) in 3.1 per cent.
>
>Small-pox in 3.1 per cent.
>
>Typhus fever in 3.1 per cent.
>
>Spinal curvature in 3.1 per cent.
>
>Somnambulism in 3.1 per cent.
>
>Scarlatina in 3.1 per cent.

The only special feature of this table is the fact that, of the cases of epilepsy under observation, convulsions at dentition were positively ascertained in 15 per cent. of the total number of cases, and in 43.7 per cent. of those having suffered from former illnesses. Here also the percentage is probably in reality greater, as it is obvious that many of the patients were ignorant as to whether or not these symptoms existed. There is no evidence that any of the other illnesses had any relation to the epilepsy.

Temperance and Intemperance.—On this head nothing definite could be ascertained. The patients either do not tell the truth, or have very elastic notions as to moderation in the use of alcoholic stimuli.

2.—EXCITING CAUSES.

To ascertain the exciting causes of epileptic seizures with exactitude is usually a matter of very great difficulty. It is simple enough when the results directly follow the cause; but this is not commonly the case. If, for example, a man, after a blow on the head (having been previously in good health) becomes suddenly seized with epileptic attacks within a few hours or days of the accident, we may fairly assume that the injury has originated or developed his illness. But should the seizure not supervene for some months or years afterwards, the external wound having in the meantime completely recovered, there remains on this question a considerable element of doubt. In the same way a patient often attributes the attacks to a fright which may have occurred weeks or months before they began; yet great care should be taken in accepting such a statement: on the other hand, it should not be utterly ignored. Again, if a person develops epilepsy after severe and prolonged domestic trouble or affliction, how are we accurately to determine the relation between the two? These difficulties render an exact method of ascertaining the exciting causes almost impossible, and this can only be approximated by a careful consideration of the entire history and circumstances of the case. Taking these into consideration, the following statements have been drawn up, in which only those conditions are recorded, where from a review of the whole case a reasonable relation was found to exist between cause and effect.

In a hundred unselected cases of epilepsy there were—

>   No apparent exciting cause in 43 per cent.
>
>   Possible exciting cause in   57 per cent.

Of the cases where a possible exciting cause was present, the following is an analysis:—

>   Blow or injury to head in   28.1 per cent.
>
>   Uterine disorder in   22.8 per cent.
>
>   Domestic trouble in   15.7 per cent.

Disease of the nervous system in 8.7 per cent.

Fright in	5.2 per cent.
Depression in	5.2 per cent.
Pregnancy in	5.2 per cent.
Mental strain in	3.5 per cent.
Sunstroke in	3.5 per cent.
Emotion in	1.7 per cent.

Thus, in no fewer than 16 per cent. of the total number of cases, and 28.1 of those in which a possible exciting cause was present, did epileptic seizures follow injuries to the head. Of the cases recorded under uterine disorders, it must be stated that these conditions were as much the accompaniments as the cause of epilepsy, the relations between the two being as follows:—

Attacks occurring at menstrual periods in	61.5 per cent.
Attacks associated with irregular menstruation in	30.7 per cent.
Attacks associated with uterine disease in	7.6 per cent.

An attempt was made in twenty-two cases to ascertain whether, in women, the age at which the epileptic attacks began had any relation to the period at which the catamenia commenced, with the following results:—

Average age at which attacks began	14.6 years
Average age at which catamenia began	14.6 years

This shows singularly enough exactly the same figures, and serves to point out, that in women, the earliest manifestation of puberty is a decided exciting cause for epileptic attacks. It must however be stated that, in the female epileptics, the attacks commenced before the age of puberty in 16.9 per cent. of their numbers. Of the 8.7 per cent. of cases included under the term "diseases of the nervous system," the epilepsy was associated with hemiplegia in all.

SYMPTOMATOLOGY.

In a hundred unselected cases of epilepsy there were—

Epilepsia gravior in	62 per cent.
Epilepsia mitior in	10 per cent.

Epilepsia gravior and mitior in 28 per cent.

1.—EPILEPSIA GRAVIOR.

Premonitory Symptoms.—In the cases in which epilepsia gravior was present there were—

    No premonitory symptoms in 34.4 per cent.

    Premonitory symptoms in   65.5 per cent.

Of those cases in which there were symptoms premonitory to the attack, there were—

    General premonitory symptoms in 47.4 per cent.

    Special Auræ in   72.8 per cent.

By *general premonitory* symptoms are understood those morbid conditions lasting for some hours or days before each attack, and of the cases under consideration in which these were present, the following is an analysis:—

    Prolonged vertigo in   46.4 per cent.

    Headache in   21.4 per cent.

    Nervousness in   14.2 per cent.

    Drowsiness in   3.5 per cent.

    Faintness in   3.5 per cent.

    Depression of spirits in   3.5 per cent.

    Cramps in   3.5 per cent.

    Numbness of extremities in 3.5 per cent.

Of the cases in which a *special aura* preceded the attack, the details are as follows (the special symptom in each case being sudden):—

    Loss of sight in   2.3 per cent.

    Loss of speech in   13.9 per cent.

    Loss of hearing in   2.3 per cent.

    General tremor in   16.2 per cent.

    Tremor of one foot in   2.3 per cent.

    Sensation in epigastrium in   6.9 per cent.

Sensation in abdomen in	4.6 per cent.
Sensation in throat in	6.9 per cent.
Sensation in left side in	2.3 per cent.
Sensation in both hands in	2.3 per cent.
Sensation in one hand in	2.3 per cent.
Violent pain in head in	2.3 per cent.
Pain in one foot in	2.3 per cent.
Sparkling sensation in eyes in	6.9 per cent.
Pumping sensation in head in	4.6 per cent.
Noises in ears in	4.6 per cent.
Diplopia in	2.3 per cent.
Contraction of one leg in	2.3 per cent.
Rotation of head in	2.3 per cent.
Distortion of face in	2.3 per cent.
Twitching of thumb in	2.3 per cent.
Spasm of eye-balls in	2.3 per cent.
Disagreeable smell in	2.3 per cent.

From these figures we find that in 34.4 per cent. of the cases of epilepsia gravior there are no special symptoms announcing the seizure, which takes place without warning of any kind; and it is especially in such cases that patients in falling, seriously injure themselves. In 65.5 per cent. there are premonitory symptoms of some kind, which indicate often many hours before the approach of an attack. Of these last 47.4 per cent. are of a general character, and in no less than 72.8 per cent. is there a distinct special aura, which in 25.4 per cent. alone precede the attack, the remainder being associated with the general premonitory symptoms.

Symptoms of the Attack.—In the cases of epilepsia gravior there were complete loss of consciousness with convulsions, lasting from five to ten minutes, and occurring at intervals, leaving no question as to the true nature of the disease, and all doubtful examples have been excluded from this collection. Attempts were made to form an analysis of the different symptoms constituting the paroxysm, but with indifferent success, and these are not here reproduced, because they are not sufficiently accurate for scientific purposes. The patient himself can give no account of what takes place. The friends around do not look upon the phenomena of the attack with the critical and philosophic eye of the physician; hence any information from them as to the part convulsed, the colour of the skin, the duration of the seizure, and so on, is extremely vague and untrustworthy. The number of cases personally observed actually during attacks is too limited to warrant any generalizations. There is, however, one important point which can be accurately demonstrated—namely, whether or not the tongue is bitten, and in the cases under observation

        The tongue was bitten in   68.8 per cent.

        The tongue was not bitten in 31.2 per cent.

Frequency of Attacks.—Only a general average of the number of attacks can be made; and in the present series the following gives an idea of the frequency of seizures in different individuals.

        Average of one or more attacks per day in   8.8 per cent.

        Average of one or more attacks per week in   31.1 per cent.

        Average of one or more attacks per month in 32.2 per cent.

        Average of one or more attacks per year in   15.5 per cent.

        At longer or more irregular intervals in   12.2 per cent.

This roughly indicates that, in the majority of cases, attacks of epilepsia gravior occur one or more times weekly or monthly. Under the last series, of attacks taking place at longer and more irregular intervals than a year, are included those cases where a few only have occurred during the lifetime of the patients.

Regularity of Attacks.—Many epileptics are attacked at regular intervals, sometimes on the same day or even hour; while others are afflicted at any time, day or night. The following indicate the proportion:—

        Attacks occur at regular intervals in   21.1 per cent.

        Attacks occur at irregular intervals in 78.8 per cent.

Time of Attack.—The following particulars alone could be definitely ascertained:—

        Attacks only during sleep in   8.8 per cent.

        Attacks only during day while awake in 8.8 per cent.

Attacks only during early morning in   15.5 per cent.

Attacks at no particular time in   55.4 per cent.

The chief feature of this observation is that in 15.5 per cent. of cases of E. Gravior the attacks always took place immediately after the patients had wakened in the morning, and this is probably due to the sudden alteration of the cerebral circulation from the sleeping to the wakeful state.

Symptoms immediately after the Attack.—The moment the attack is over sometimes the patient is in his usual condition, and feels no ill effects from the paroxysm. More commonly, however, he suffers from various symptoms, the chief of which, and their relative frequency, is as follows:—

Return to usual condition in 12.2 per cent.

Drowsy in   66.6 per cent.

Confused in   14.4 per cent.

Stupid in   13.3 per cent.

Irritable in   14.4 per cent.

Excitable in   3.3 per cent.

Vertigo in   13.3 per cent.

Headache in   41.1 per cent.

The above conditions may last from an hour to several days.

Present condition, or state between the Attacks.—It is impossible to enter minutely into the actual physical and mental health of all the epileptic cases under notice, but the following statement gives a sketch of some of the more important conditions associated with the disease, and the frequency with which they occur. In the inter-paroxysmal state the condition of the patients were—

Healthy in every respect in   17.7 per cent.

With some abnormal peculiarity in 82.2 per cent.

General health good in   75.5 per cent.

General health impaired in   24.4 per cent.

Robust in	66.6 per cent.
Not robust in	33.3 per cent.
Intelligence intact in	74.4 per cent.
Intelligence impaired in	25.5 per cent.
Loss of memory in	58.8 per cent.
No loss of memory in	41.1 per cent.
Stupid in	16.6 per cent.
Dull in	31.1 per cent.
Irritable in	25.4 per cent.
Frequent headaches in	41.1 per cent.
Frequent vertigo in	22.2 per cent.
Nervous in	21.1 per cent.
Special diseases in	21.1 per cent.

Of the 21.1 per cent. under the heading of special diseases, there were—

Hemiplegia in	6.6 per cent.
Paralysis of seventh nerve in	1.1 per cent.
Impediment of speech in	1.1 per cent.
Cicatrix over sciatic nerve in	1.1 per cent.
Idiot in	1.1 per cent.
Anæmia in	5.5 per cent.
Phthisis in	2.2 per cent.
Confirmed dyspepsia in	1.1 per cent.

From these details it is evident that epilepsy is not of necessity associated with impairment of the physical or mental health. On the contrary, we find that in 17.7 per cent. of the patients there was apparently no flaw of any kind in their constitutions, which were absolutely normal, with the exception of the periodic seizures. In no less than 75.5 per cent. was the general health good, and in 66.6 per cent. the patients were robust and vigorous. At the same time the health was markedly impaired in 24.4 per cent., and the sufferers were of delicate or weak habit in 33.3 per cent. The main fact, however, to be observed is that, in the majority of cases of epilepsy, the general health and vigour of the patient is not deteriorated. In the same way, the intellectual capacities are not of necessity affected. In 74.4 per cent. the intelligence is recorded as not seriously impaired; and in 41.1 per cent. the memory as good. On the other hand, the mental faculties were markedly deficient in 25.5 per cent.; the patients were dull and slow in 31.1 per cent.; and in more than half, or 58.8 per cent., was there evidence of loss of memory. Another frequent symptom is repeated and constant headache, which, in the present series of cases, existed in 41.1 per cent.

2.—EPILEPSIA MITIOR.

This occurred altogether in 38 per cent. of the total number of cases. In these it occurred—

> By itself in 26.3 per cent.
>
> Associated with E. Gravior in 73.6 per cent.

In all, the usual characteristics of the *petit mal* presented themselves; there being temporary loss of consciousness, sometimes with slight spasms, but without true convulsion, biting of the tongue, &c.

Frequency of Attacks.—The rough average frequency of attacks, as estimated in the cases under consideration, was as follows:—

> 20 to 30 attacks per day in 3.7 per cent.
>
> 10 to 20 attacks per day in 7.4 per cent.
>
> 5 to 10 attacks per day in 14.8 per cent.
>
> 1 to 5 attacks per day in 40.7 per cent.
>
> 1 or more attacks per week in 22.2 per cent.
>
> 1 or more attacks per month in 7.4 per cent.
>
> At rarer intervals in 3.7 per cent.

Thus when epilepsia mitior exists, in the majority of cases the attacks are of daily occurrence.

Loss of consciousness, as ascertained in a series of cases, was

Complete in 48.3 per cent.

Partial in   51.6 per cent.

Premonitory Symptoms.—These are not, as a rule, so well marked in epilepsia mitior as in E. Gravior; but frequently the aura is quite as distinctly appreciated. In the 28 per cent. of cases in which E. Mitior is associated with E. Gravior, the aura was apparently the same in both. Of the 10 per cent. cases of E. Mitior occurring by itself, the following is the record:—

No aura in	20 per cent.
Sensation in epigastrium in	20 per cent.
Loss of speech in	10 per cent.
Violent pain in head in	10 per cent.
Tingling of extremities in	10 per cent.
Choking sensation in	10 per cent.
Hallucination in	10 per cent.
Vertigo in	10 per cent.

The number of cases in E. Mitior is too limited to warrant further generalization.

FOOTNOTES:

[A] Reprinted from the "British Medical Journal" of March 15 & 22, 1879.

II.

AN INQUIRY

INTO THE

ACTION OF THE BROMIDES ON

EPILEPTIC ATTACKS.[B]

Bromide of potassium is generally recognised as the most effective anti-epileptic remedy we at present possess. There exists, however, great difference of opinion as to its method of administration and to the amount of benefit which we may expect from its use. Some physicians who employ the drug after one method come to totally different conclusions as to its efficacy from those who use another. Many believe the remedy to be only useful in certain forms of the disease, and to be very uncertain and imperfect in its action. Others, again, maintain that it is positively injurious to the general health of the patient. These and other unsettled points the following inquiry attempts to make clear.

Epilepsy, like all other chronic diseases, presents great difficulties in scientifically estimating the exact value of any particular remedy; and unless the investigation of the subject is approached with the strictest impartiality, and observations made with rigid accuracy, we are liable to fall into the most misleading fallacies. I believe that these are to be avoided, and facts arrived at, however laborious it may be to the experimenter and wearisome to the student, only by the careful observation and elaborate record of an extensive series of cases. If, in epilepsy, the disease, from its prolonged duration, its doubtful causation and pathology, its serious complications and the many other mysterious circumstances connected with it, offers almost unsurmountable difficulties to any definite and uniform method of treatment and the systematic estimation of the same, its symptoms furnish us with tolerably accurate data upon which to base our observations. The attacks, although only symptoms, may be practically considered as representing the disease, as in the large majority of cases, in proportion as these are frequent and severe, so much the more serious is the affection. The influence of the bromides on these paroxysms is taken in the following inquiry to represent the action of these drugs on the epileptic state.

Before proceeding to detail the facts arrived at, it is necessary briefly to state the method of procedure adopted in treatment. Each case in succession, and without selection, which was pronounced to be epilepsy (all doubtful cases being eliminated), was considered as a subject suitable for experiment. The general circumstances of the individual were studied; his diet, hygienic surroundings, habits, and so on, if faulty, were, when practicable, improved. The bromides were then ordered, and taken without intermission for periods which will subsequently be detailed. The minimum quantity for an adult, to begin with, was thirty grains three times a day, the first dose half an hour before rising in the morning, the second in the middle of the day on an empty stomach, and the third at bedtime. This was continued for a fortnight, and if with success, was persevered with, according to circumstances, for a period varying from two to six months. If, on the other hand, the attacks were not materially diminished in frequency, the dose was immediately increased by ten grains at a time till the paroxysms were arrested. In this way as much as from sixty to eighty grains have been administered three times daily, and, with one or two isolated exceptions to be afterwards pointed out, I have met with no case of epilepsy which altogether resisted the influence of these large doses; and, moreover, I have never seen any really serious symptoms of poisoning or injury to the general health ensue in consequence. Sometimes these quantities of the drugs have been taken for many months with advantage; but as a rule it is preferable, when possible, after a few weeks gradually to diminish the dose and endeavour to secure that amount which, while it does not injuriously affect the general condition of the patient, serves to keep the epileptic attacks in subjection. The form of prescription to begin with in an adult has been as follows:—

- ℞ Pot. bromid., gr. xv.
    - Ammon. bromid., gr. xv.
    - Sp. ammon. aromat., m. xx.
    - Infus. quassia, ad ℨj

M. Ft. haust. ter die, sumendus.

According to the age of the patient so must the dose be regulated; at the same time, children bear the drug very well. The average quantity to begin with for a child of ten or twelve years has been twenty grains thrice daily.

In this manner I have personally treated about two hundred cases, and in all of these most careful records have been kept, not only of their past history, present condition, etc., but of their progress during observation. All these, however, are not available for the present inquiry. It is necessary in order to judge of the true effect of a drug in epilepsy that the patient should be under its influence continuously for a certain period of time. Now, a large number of patients, especially amongst the working classes, cannot or will not be induced to persevere in the prolonged treatment necessary in so chronic a disease. They either weary of the monotony of drinking physic, especially if, as is often the case, they are relieved for the time, or other circumstances prevent their carrying out the regimen to its full extent. The minimum time I have fixed as a test for judging the influence of the bromides on epileptic seizures is six months, and the maximum in my own experience extends to four years.[C] All other cases have been eliminated. I have arranged this experience in the form of tables for reference, in which will be seen at a glance—*1st*, the average number of attacks per month in each case prior to treatment; *2nd*, the average number of attacks per month after treatment; and *3rd*, in the event of these being fewer than one seizure per month, the total number during the last six months of treatment.

TABLE I.—*Sixty Cases of Epilepsy, showing Results of Treatment by the Bromides during a Period of from 6 Months to 1 Year.*

No. of Case.	Average number attacks per month *before* treatment.	Average number attacks per month *after* treatment.	Number of attacks during six months of treatment.
1	900	60	—
2	600	5	—
3	600	90	—
4	450	12	—
5	300	2	—
6	240	90	—
7	180	60	—
8	150	5	—
9	150	8	—
10	150	7	—
11	120	3	—
12	120	120	—
13	90	3	—
14	90	9	—
15	70	20	—

16	60	4	—
17	60	6	—
18	60	90	—
19	30	7	—
20	30	1	—
21	30	2	—
22	30	10	—
23	16	8	—
24	16	2	—
25	12	4	—
26	12	12	—
27	12	3	—
28	8	0	0
29	8	2	—
30	8	1	—
31	8	1	—
32	8	—	4
33	8	1	—
34	8	4	—
35	6	0	0
36	5	—	5
37	5	0	0
38	4	2	—
39	4	1	—
40	4	1	—
41	4	1	—
42	4	—	2
43	4	—	3
44	2	—	3
45	2	—	2

46	2	—	1
47	2	—	1
48	2	—	4
49	2	—	1
50	2	—	2
51	1	0	0
52	1	—	2
53	1	0	0
54	1	1	—
55	1	0	0
56	1	0	0
57	1	—	1
58	1	—	1
59	1	—	1
60	1	150	—

TABLE II.—*Thirty-two Cases of Epilepsy, showing Results of Treatment by the Bromides during a period of from 1 to 2 Years.*

No. of Case.	Average number attacks per month *before* treatment.	Average number attacks per month *after* treatment.	Number of attacks during six months of treatment.
1	900	60	—
2	600	120	—
3	300	30	—
4	180	60	—
5	150	—	2
6	150	1	—
7	90	9	—
8	90	15	—
9	60	2	—
10	6	—	4
11	30	—	1

12	30	4	—
13	30	2	—
14	30	3	—
15	16	—	8
16	12	3	—
17	8	0	0
18	8	—	3
19	8	—	4
20	8	—	1
21	8	—	10
22	6	—	1
23	4	—	4
24	4	—	4
25	4	2	—
26	2	—	1
27	2	—	2
28	2	—	2
29	1	0	0
30	1	0	0
31	1	—	3
32	1	—	3

TABLE III.—*Seventeen Cases of Epilepsy, showing Results of Treatment by the Bromides during a Period of from Two to Three Years.*

No. of Case.	Average number attacks per month *before* treatment.	Average number attacks per month *after* treatment.	Number of attacks during six months of treatment.
1	600	60	—
2	300	15	—
3	60	—	8
4	30	—	4

No.	Average number attacks per month before treatment.	Average number attacks per month after treatment.	Number of attacks during six months of treatment.
5	30	—	8
6	30	—	2
7	16	2	—
8	12	—	8
9	8	—	2
10	8	—	1
11	8	—	3
12	4	—	1
13	4	1	—
14	4	6	—
15	1	0	0
16	1	0	0
17	1	—	3

TABLE IV.—*Eight Cases of Epilepsy, showing the Results of Treatment by the Bromides during a period of from Three to Four Years.*

No. of Case.	Average number attacks per month *before* treatment.	Average number attacks per month *after* treatment.	Number of attacks during six months of treatment.
1	300	3	—
2	60	1	—
3	60	4	—
4	30	1	—
5	16	—	10
6	12	—	3
7	8	0	0
8	1	0	0

These four tables consist of all the characteristic cases of epilepsy which came under notice, without selection of any kind, all being included, no matter what their form or severity, their age, complication with organic disease, etc. In analyzing this miscellaneous series, the chief fact to be noticed, whether the period of treatment has been limited to six months or extended to four years, is the remarkable effect of treatment upon the number of the epileptic seizures. Of the total 117 cases, in 14, or about 12.1

per cent., the attacks were entirely arrested during the whole period of treatment. In 97, or about 83.3 per cent., the monthly number of seizures was diminished. In 3, or about 2.3 per cent., there was no change either for better or worse; and in 3, or about 2.3 per cent., the attacks were more frequent after treatment.

With regard to the fourteen cases which were free from attacks during treatment, it cannot, of course, be maintained that all of these were cured in the strict sense of the term. It is probable that if any of them discontinued the medicine the seizures would return. Still, the results are such as to encourage a hope that if the bromides are persevered with, and the attacks arrested for a sufficiently long period, a permanent result might be anticipated. Even should no such ultimate object be realized, it is obvious that an agent which can, during its administration, completely cut short the distressing epileptic paroxysms, without injuriously affecting the mental or bodily health, is of immense importance. Take, for example, cases 7 and 8 of Table IV., where, prior to treatment, in the one case eight fits a month, and in the other one, were completely arrested during a period of nearly four years. The experience of physicians agrees in considering that the danger of epilepsy, both to mind and body, is in great part directly proportionate to the severity of its symptoms. If these latter can be completely arrested, even should we be compelled to continue the treatment, if this is without injury to the patient, it is as close an approach to cure as we can ever expect to arrive at by therapeutic means. The permanent nature of the improvement, and the possibility of subsequent discontinuance of the bromides without return of the disease, is a question I shall not enter into, as my own personal experience is not yet sufficiently extended to be able to form a practical opinion. A satisfactory solution of this problem could only be made after a life-long private practice, or by the accumulated experience of many observers. With hospital patients such is almost impossible, as they are lost sight of, especially if they recover.

Of the total 117 cases which compose the tables, we find that in no less than 97 were the attacks beneficially influenced by the bromides. In the different cases this improvement varies in degree, but in most of them it is very considerable—for example, Nos. 2, 5, 8, 11, 20, in Table I; Nos. 5, 6, 11, 15, in Table II; Nos. 3, 4, 5, 6, in Table III; and all the cases in Table IV. In these and others the attacks, if not actually arrested, were so enormously curtailed, both in number and severity, in comparison to what existed before treatment, as to constitute a most important change in the condition of the patient. In those cases in which improvement was not so well marked, in many it was most decided, and in frequent instances caused life, which had become a burden to the patient and his friends, to be bearable.

Of the total number of cases, in 3 the administration of the bromides had no effect whatever in diminishing the attacks, and in 3 others the number of seizures was greater after treatment than before. Whether in these last this circumstance was the result of the drug, or due to some co-incident augmentation of the disease itself, I cannot decide, but am inclined to believe in the latter as the explanation.

After a consideration of these facts it is difficult to understand why most physicians look upon epilepsy as an *opprobrium medicinæ*, and of all diseases as one of the least amenable to treatment, and the despair of the therapeutist. For example, Nothnagel, one of the most recent and representative authorities on the subject, in speaking of the treatment of epilepsy, says, "Many remedies and methods of treatment have isolated successes to show, but nothing is to be depended on; nothing can, on a careful discrimination of cases, afford a sure prospect of recovery, or even improvement." Such a statement indicates either an imperfect method of treatment, or that in Germany epilepsy is more intractable than in this country, as a "careful discrimination" of the above cases affords a "sure prospect of improvement" and a reasonable one of recovery. That a critical spirit and healthy scepticism should exist regarding the vague and imperfect accounts of the efficacy of various drugs in disease is, I believe, necessary to arrive at the truth; at the same time, we must not refuse to credit evidence sufficiently based on observation and experiment. The above collection of cases are facts, carefully and laboriously recorded, and not originally intended for the purpose which they at present fulfil. Having been brought up in the belief that epilepsy was one of the most intractable of diseases, no one is more surprised than myself at the readiness with which it responds to treatment. So far, then, from this affection being the despair of the profession, I believe that of all chronic nervous diseases it is the one most amenable to treatment by drugs, resulting, if not in complete cure, in great amelioration of the symptoms which practically constitute the disease.

An important consideration next arises. Assuming that practically the treatment in all cases is alike, are there any special circumstances which explain why some patients should have no attacks while under the influence of the drugs, while others are only relieved; why some—though the number is very small—should receive no benefit, and others have a larger number of attacks after treatment? On a careful examination of all the clinical facts of each case, no explanation can be found, the same form of attack, the same complications and circumstances, occupying each group. For example, one of those who had no attacks during treatment was a woman who had been afflicted with epilepsy for eighteen years, of a severe form, with general convulsions, biting tongue, etc. Another was a very delicate, nervous woman, who suffered, in addition to the seizures, from pulmonary and laryngeal phthisis, who came of a family impregnated with epilepsy, and whose intellect was greatly impaired. By far the largest class are those benefited by treatment, and these comprehend every species of case, chronic and recent, complicated, inherited, in the old and young, and so on; yet the most careful analysis fails to discover why some should be more amenable to treatment than others, or give any indication which might be useful in prognosis. Neither does a study of the few cases which the bromides did not affect, or those which increased in severity under their influence, throw any light upon the subject, as some of these latter gave no indications beforehand of their unfortunate termination, and in none of them was there any serious complication or special departure from good mental or bodily health.

Another point must be noted, although there is no statistical method of demonstrating the fact, namely, that in those cases in which the attacks were not completely arrested, but only diminished in number, those seizures which remained were frequently greatly modified in character while the patient was under the influence of the bromides. These were less severe, and characterized by the patients as "slight," while formerly they were "strong." This by itself often proves of great service, as, instead of a severe convulsive fit, in which the patient severely injures himself, bites his tongue, etc., he has what he calls a "sensation," in other words, an abortive attack.

Having considered the general effects of the bromides on a series of unselected cases, we now proceed to investigate whether any particular form of the disease, or any special circumstances connected with the patient or his surroundings, have any influence in modifying the results of treatment. The following table shows epilepsy divided into its two chief forms, namely, E. Gravior and E. Mitior. By the former is understood the ordinary severe attack, with loss of consciousness and convulsions; the latter is the slighter and very temporary seizure, of loss of consciousness, but without convulsions.

TABLE V.—*Showing Results of Treatment by the Bromides in*—1. *Epilepsia Gravior*, *and* 2. *Epilepsia Mitior.*

No. of Case.	Average number attacks per month *before* treatment.	Average number attacks per month *after* treatment.	Number of attacks during six months of treatment.
1. *Epilepsia Gravior.*			
1	600	5	—
2	450	12	—

3	249	90	—
4	180	60	—
5	120	3	—
6	60	1	—
7	60	6	—
8	30	—	8
9	30	4	—
10	30	12	—
11	23	1	—
12	16	2	—
13	12	—	4
14	12	3	—
15	12	10	—
16	8	0	0
17	8	—	4
18	8	1	—
19	8	4	—
20	8	2	—
21	6	—	1
22	5	—	5
23	5	0	0
24	4	—	2
25	4	1	—
26	4	2	—
27	2	—	1
28	2	—	1
29	2	—	1
30	2	—	1
31	2	—	2
32	2	—	2

33	1	0	0
34	1	0	0
35	1	0	0
36	1	0	0
37	1	0	0
38	1	0	0
39	1	—	1
40	1	—	1
41	1	—	1
42	1	—	1
43	1	—	2
44	1	—	4
45	1	—	2
46	1	1	—
47	1	150	—

2. *Epilepsia Mitior.*

1	900	60	—
2	600	60	—
3	300	3	—
4	150	1	—
5	150	7	—
6	120	120	—
7	90	9	—
8	90	3	—
9	60	15	—
10	60	90	—
11	13	—	2
12	16	—	4
13	16	—	8
14	8	—	3

15	8	—	3
16	4	—	1
17	4	6	—
18	1	—	4

Of 47 cases of E. Major, we find that in 8 there were no attacks during the whole period of treatment, in 1 there was no improvement, in 1 the attacks were augmented after treatment, and in 37 there was marked and varying diminution of the seizures. Of 18 cases of E. Mitior there was no case where the attacks were wholly suspended, in 1 there was no improvement, in 2 the attacks were increased, and in 15 they were diminished in number by treatment. This is scarcely a fair comparison between the two forms, as the numbers are so unequal; but cases of uncomplicated E. Mitior are not common, being generally associated with the graver form, which combined cases are not inserted in this table. It is generally asserted in books that the non-convulsive form is much more intractable than the other, but the above table proves the contrary, as, for example, in Nos. 3, 4, 11, 12. It is true that the results do not appear so complete or striking in E. Mitior as in E. Gravior, but then it must be remembered that the number of cases is more limited, and the number of attacks originally much greater. In short, the table shows that if treatment does not completely avert the attacks of E. Mitior, it greatly diminishes their frequency.

TABLE VI.—*Showing Effects of Treatment by the Bromides in Epilepsy. 1. Diurnal Form; 2. Nocturnal Form.*

No. of Case.	Average number attacks per month *before* treatment.	Average number attacks per month *after* treatment.	Number of attacks during six months of treatment.
1. *Diurnal Form.*			
1	300	3	—
2	90	9	—
3	60	6	—
4	30	—	8
5	24	1	—
6	16	—	8
7	12	—	4
8	8	—	3

9	8	—	4
10	4	1	—
11	2	—	1
12	1	0	0
13	1	0	0
14	1	0	0
15	1	—	1
2. *Nocturnal Form.*			
1	60	1	—
2	16	—	4
3	8	2	—
4	2	—	1
5	4	—	2
6	1	—	—
7	1	150	—

Another variety of epilepsy is that which is characterized by the time at which the attacks occur. In the large majority of cases these take place both while the patient is awake and when he is asleep. I have, unfortunately, no observations to offer as to the effects of treatment on the diurnal or nocturnal attacks in patients suffering from both. The preceding table shows the result of treatment in 15 cases in which the attacks occurred only while the patient was awake, and in 7 cases where they took place only while he was asleep.

Of 15 cases of the purely diurnal form, we find that in 3 there was a total cessation of attacks during treatment, and in all the others there was diminution in their number. Of the 7 nocturnal cases, in none were the seizures entirely arrested, in 1 the attacks increased in number after treatment, and the remainder were relieved to a greater or less extent. Here, again, our numbers are small, and therefore difficult to found any definite principle upon; still there is enough to show that, contrary to the opinion expressed by most authorities, the nocturnal form of epilepsy appears to be as amenable to relief as the diurnal variety.

The next point for consideration is the question whether the fact of the epilepsy being hereditary or not makes any difference in the results of treatment by the bromides. In the following table all the cases with a perfectly sound family history are placed in the first part, and the second includes those in which either epilepsy or insanity could be proved to exist in any near relation.

Thus in 39 cases with a perfectly sound family history, in 3 the attacks were totally arrested during treatment, in 2 there was no improvement, in 2 there was increase of seizures after treatment, and in the remainder there was diminution of the fits. In 18 cases, where at least one near relation suffered from either epilepsy or insanity, in 3 the attacks were arrested, in 1 they were increased, and in the remainder diminished. In short, from a review of the details of the table, it does not appear that the fact of the disease being inherited, or of its existing in other members of the family, makes any difference to the benefit we may expect to derive from treatment.

TABLE VII.—*Showing Effects of Treatment by the Bromides in Epilepsy.* 1. *Non-Hereditary Cases*, 2. *Hereditary Cases.*

No. of Case.	Average number attacks per month *before* treatment.	Average number attacks per month *after* treatment.	Number of attacks during six months of treatment.
1. *Non-Hereditary Cases.*			
1	600	5	—
2	600	60	—
3	450	12	—
4	240	90	—
5	300	3	—
6	150	7	—
7	120	3	—
8	120	120	—
9	150	1	—
10	70	20	—
11	60	6	—
12	60	90	—
13	60	1	—
14	30	12	—
15	90	3	—

16	30	—	2
17	16	—	4
18	16	2	—
19	8	0	0
20	8	2	—
21	8	—	3
22	8	4	—
23	6	—	1
24	5	0	0
25	5	—	5
26	4	2	—
27	4	1	—
28	2	—	2
29	2	—	1
30	2	1	—
31	2	—	2
32	1	0	0
33	1	—	2
34	1	—	4
35	1	1	—
36	1	—	1
37	1	—	1
38	1	—	1
39	1	150	—
2. *Hereditary Cases.*			
1	900	60	—
2	180	60	—
3	90	9	—
4	24	1	—
5	16	—	8

No. of Case	Avg. before	Avg. after	No. during six months
6	12	—	4
7	12	3	—
8	8	1	—
9	8	—	3
10	8	—	4
11	4	—	2
12	4	6	—
13	2	—	1
14	2	—	1
15	1	0	0
16	1	0	0
17	1	0	0
18	4	—	1

The next table attempts to show whether or not the age of the patient when he came under observation has any effect in modifying the action of the bromides, or whether it assists us prognosing the probable result.

A survey of this table shows in general terms that the age of the patient is neither an assistance nor impediment to the successful action of the bromides in the treatment of epilepsy. Whatever the age may be, whether in a young child or in an old person, the average of beneficial effects appears to be the same. At first sight it would seem as if treatment would be more successful in the young; but it is not so, as the two cases in the table over fifty years of age received as much average benefit as any of the others.

TABLE VIII.—*Showing Effects of Treatment by the Bromides in Epilepsy at Different Ages.* 1. *Under 15 Years;* 2. *Between 15 and 30 Years;* 3. *Between 30 and 50 Years;* 4. *Over 50 Years.*

No. of Case.	Average number attacks per month *before* treatment.	Average number attacks per month *after* treatment.	Number of attacks during six months of treatment.
1. *Under 15 Years.*			
1	900	60	—
2	600	5	—
3	600	60	—
4	450	12	—

5	240	90	—
6	180	60	—
7	150	7	—
8	30	4	—
9	8	0	0
10	8	—	3
11	4	6	—
12	4	2	—
13	2	—	1
14	1	150	—

2. *Between 15 and 30 Years.*

1	300	3	—
2	150	7	—
3	120	3	—
4	120	120	—
5	90	3	—
6	60	1	—
7	60	6	—
8	60	90	—
9	16	—	4
10	16	—	8
11	16	2	—
12	12	—	4
13	8	1	4
14	8	2	—
15	8	4	—
16	70	20	—
17	5	0	0
18	4	—	2
19	4	1	—

20	4	1	—
21	2	—	2
22	2	—	1
23	2	—	1
24	2	—	2
25	1	0	0
26	1	0	0
27	1	0	0
28	1	—	1
29	1	—	2
30	1	—	4
31	1	1	—

3. *Between 30 and 50 Years.*

1	30	—	2
2	30	—	12
3	12	3	—
4	8	1	—
5	8	—	3
6	5	—	5
7	2	—	2
8	1	0	0
9	1	—	1
10	1	—	1

4. *Over 50 Years.*

1	30	—	8
2	24	1	—

Does the fact of the disease being recent or chronic affect the prognosis of treatment? This will be seen by the following table, in which the length of time that the disease has existed is divided into four periods, namely—1, those cases in which the attacks first began less than a year before treatment was commenced; 2, those in which they had begun from one to five years before; 3, those in which they began from five to ten years before; and, 4, those in which the disease had existed for over ten years.

TABLE IX.—*Showing Effects of Treatment by the Bromides in Epilepsy in Recent and Chronic Cases. 1. Under 1 Year; 2. From 1 to 5 Years; 3. From 5 to 10 Years; 4. Over 10 Years.*

No. of Case.	Average number attacks per month *before* treatment.	Average number attacks per month *after* treatment.	Number of attacks during six months of treatment.
1. *Under 1 Year.*			
1	600	60	—
2	60	6	—
3	8	—	3
4	5	0	0
5	4	—	2
6	4	2	—
7	2	—	1
8	2	—	1
9	2	—	2
2. *From 1 to 5 Years.*			
1	600	5	—
2	240	90	—
3	180	60	—
4	90	3	—
5	30	—	2
6	30	—	8
7	30	12	—
8	16	—	8
9	12	3	—
10	8	0	0
11	150	7	—
12	8	2	—
13	6	1	—

14	4	—	1
15	2	—	1
16	2	—	2
17	1	0	0
18	1	0	0
19	1	—	1
20	1	1	—
21	1	150	—

3. *From 5 to 10 Years.*

1	450	12	—
2	300	3	—
3	900	60	—
4	90	9	—
5	60	1	—
6	30	4	—
7	16	2	—
8	8	—	4
9	8	—	3
10	8	1	—
11	4	1	—
12	3	1	—
13	1	—	1
14	1	—	1
15	1	—	2

4. *Over 10 Years.*

1	150	1	—
2	120	3	—
3	120	120	—
4	70	20	—
5	60	90	—

6	16	—	4
7	12	—	4
8	8	4	—
9	5	—	5
10	1	0	0
11	1	0	0
12	1	—	4

In this table we observe very singular results in the treatment of this remarkable disease. In most ailments, the longer they have existed and the more chronic they are, the more difficult and imperfect is the prospect of recovery. This does not appear to hold good in the case of epilepsy. For when we analyze the above table we find that the results, on an average, are as satisfactory in those cases in which the disease has existed over ten years as in those which began less than one year before the patient came under observation. For example, we find in section 4 of Table IX. 12 cases in which epilepsy had existed for over ten years prior to treatment; of these, in 2 the attacks were completely arrested, in 1 there was no improvement, in 1 the attacks were increased, and in the remainder the seizures were as beneficially modified as in the other sections. Thus it would seem that we are not to be deterred from treating cases of epilepsy, however chronic they may be, as the results appear to be as good in modifying the attacks in old, as in recent cases.

TABLE X.—*Showing Effects of Treatment by the Bromides in Epilepsy—1. In Healthy Persons; 2. In Diseased Persons.*

No. of Case.	Average number attacks per month *before* treatment.	Average number attacks per month *after* treatment.	Number of attacks during six months of treatment.
1. *Healthy Persons.*			
1	900	60	—
2	600	60	—
3	150	7	—
4	150	1	—
5	120	3	—
6	90	9	—
7	70	20	—

8	60	1	—
9	60	5	—
10	60	90	—
11	30	—	2
12	30	—	8
13	30	12	—
14	16	0	0
15	16	2	—
16	16	—	4
17	12	3	—
18	8	2	—
19	8	0	0
20	8	—	3
21	8	—	4
22	8	4	—
23	4	2	—
24	4	1	—
25	4	2	—
26	2	—	1
27	2	—	2
28	2	—	1
29	2	—	1
30	2	—	2
31	2	—	1
32	1	0	0
33	1	—	2
34	1	1	—
35	1	0	0
36	1	0	0
37	1	—	1

38	1	—	1
39	1	—	1
40	1	1	4
41	1	150	—
2. *Diseased Persons.*			
1	450	12	—
2	300	3	—
3	240	90	—
4	180	60	—
5	90	3	—
6	60	6	—
7	24	1	—
8	12	—	4
9	8	—	3
10	8	1	—
11	6	—	1
12	5	—	5
13	4	—	1
14	4	6	—
15	1	0	0

Another important question arises: Does the general health of the patient in any way influence the effects of treatment? In the preceding table those cases are collected in section 1 whose general health was to all appearances robust and free from disease. In section 2. are those in which organic disease could be demonstrated, or in which the condition of the patient was evidently unfavourable.

Here, again, a consideration of the table demonstrates that the condition of the general health has no influence on the successful progress of treatment, as those cases under the head of diseased persons made apparently as satisfactory progress as those in a perfectly robust condition regarding their epileptic symptoms.

As a specimen, the following table shows the result in those cases complicated with a permanent lesion of a motor part of the brain, namely, hemiplegia, and of an intellectual portion, in the shape of idiocy:—

TABLE XI.—*Showing effects of Treatment by the Bromides in Epilepsy complicated with*—1. *Hemiplegia;* 2. *Idiocy.*

No. of Case.	Average number attacks per month *before* treatment.	Average number attacks per month *after* treatment.	Number of attacks during six months of treatment.
1. *Hemiplegia.*			
1	450	12	—
2	240	90	—
3	30	4	—
4	24	1	—
5	8	—	3
6	8	1	—
7	4	6	—
2. *Idiocy.*			
1	180	60	—
2	120	120	—
3	60	6	—
4	30	4	—
5	4	6	—

Here it may be observed that of 7 cases complicated with hemiplegia, in 1 the attacks were increased after treatment, but all the others were relieved in average proportion. Of the 5 cases in idiots, in 1 there was no improvement, in 1 the attacks were subsequently augmented, and in the others there was improvement. The numbers are far too limited to found any reliable dictum upon; at the same time, it must be admitted that while epilepsy complicated with these grave lesions is perfectly amenable to treatment, this table serves to show that the proportion of non-success is comparatively large.

It has been stated before that no attempt would be made in this paper to prove that epilepsy was curable by therapeutic means. Its aim has been to show the effects of the bromides on the attacks or symptoms of that disease. It is common to hear it remarked, as if this were of no importance, "You only arrest the fits, but you do not know, and cannot cure, the original lesion. You do not go to the fountain-head of the disease, but simply relieve its results." In reply, I would ask, Of what disease do we know the ultimate nature any better than that of epilepsy? and if we did, how would that assist us in treating it? What drug in our pharmacopœia cures any single disease, or do other than, by attacking and relieving symptoms, leave nature to remove the morbid lesion? Even quinine, to which therapeutists triumphantly point, only arrests certain paroxysms until time removes the poison from the blood, as it does in most malarious affections. So far from being a small matter, I believe there are few, if any, drugs at our disposal which can be demonstrated to have a more beneficial action in the treatment of disease than that of the bromides, in epilepsy. Besides, I decline to admit the statement that complete recovery does not follow their administration. Various authors have reported cases, and that these are rare is due to reasons stated before, and chiefly on account of the long period of treatment necessary to ensure success.

This inquiry may be summed up in the following general conclusions:—

1. In 12.1 per cent. of epileptics the attacks were completely arrested during the whole period of treatment by the bromides.
2. In 83.3 per cent. the attacks were greatly diminished both in number and severity.
3. In 2.3 per cent. the treatment had no apparent effect.
4. In 2.3 per cent. the number of attacks was augmented during the period of treatment.
5. The form of the disease, whether it was inherited or not, whether complicated or not, recent or chronic, in the young or in the old, in healthy or diseased persons, appeared in no way to influence treatment, the success being nearly in the *same ratio* under all these conditions.

FOOTNOTES:

[B] Reprinted from the "Edinburgh Medical Journal" for February and March, 1881.

[C] For an extended experience, see the next paper.

III.

AN INQUIRY

INTO THE

EFFECTS OF THE PROLONGED

ADMINISTRATION OF THE BROMIDES

IN EPILEPSY.[D]

The present inquiry is the result of an experience of 300 cases of epilepsy treated by myself with the bromides of potassium and ammonium. In all of these the clinical facts, as well as the progress of the malady, were carefully studied and recorded. The effects of the administration of these remedies on epileptic seizures I have already investigated and demonstrated in a somewhat elaborate series of observations.[E] Further experience has confirmed the correctness of the general propositions then arrived at, so that they need not again be elaborated in detail.

At present it is proposed to direct attention to the effects of the prolonged administration of large doses of the bromides, and to attempt to ascertain if, while arresting or diminishing the frequency and severity of the paroxysmal symptoms, they beneficially influence the disease itself, or in any way injuriously modify the constitution of the patient. On this subject much difference of opinion and misconception prevail. It is well known that the injudicious use of the drugs leads to certain physiological phenomena which are comprised under the term "bromism." It is also generally believed that the physical and mental depression resulting from their prolonged toxic effects constitutes a condition worse than the malady for which they are exhibited. One of the objects of this article is to question the accuracy of this assertion, a true apprehension of which is the more important when we reflect how universal is this method of treatment, and the deterrent effect it exercises upon epileptic attacks. The task, like other therapeutic inquiries—especially those connected with chronic disease—is a difficult one, there being innumerable pitfalls of error between us and a sound scientific conclusion. These, however, may, I believe, in great measure be surmounted by the accumulation of facts laboriously and accurately recorded, by the intelligent study of their details, and the impartial and logical deductions which may be drawn from the data supplied. The value of a therapeutic inquiry depends, not upon the opinions and undigested experience of individuals, or by the narration of isolated cases, but upon the indisputable proofs resulting from the unbiassed analysis of a large series of accurately observed and unselected examples. The solution of the problem, if complex in all clinical affections, is especially so in epilepsy. Although the symptoms of this disease have been recognised from the earliest ages, our knowledge of its essential nature is as yet shrouded in mystery. The etiology and pathology are practically undetermined. The phenomena are not only due to a varied series of morbid conditions, but may assume a multitude of forms and degrees of severity, which may be, on the one hand, of the briefest duration, or, on the other, of a life-long permanence. The symptoms may comprise not only a diversity of physical ailments, but intellectual disturbances of the most terrible import. The malady may attack not only many whose systems are predisposed to disease, but those of the most robust constitution and with a healthy, family history. The consequences of the disorder may be comparatively innocuous, but in other circumstances may be attended with the most disastrous effects on mind and body and even on life itself. In a disease presenting such an intricate and uncertain course, it is obviously a task of the utmost difficulty to scientifically estimate the exact value of any therapeutic measures which may be adopted for its relief. The effects on one symptom, and that the most prominent, can, however, be accurately determined—namely, the paroxysmal seizures, which are definite and computable; and this has already been accomplished with tolerable precision.[F] On the influence of the bromides on the disease itself, or on the epileptic state, we have less accurate information. In attempting to throw some light on this subject, two preliminary considerations must be recognised—1st, the physiological actions of the drug on the healthy subject; and 2nd, the inter-paroxysmal symptoms of the epileptic constitution.

1. Medicinal doses of the bromides produce in healthy persons a general diminution of nervous energy. They act as a sedative, and thus dispose to repose and sleep. If they are excessive in quantity and long continued, especially in those susceptible to their action, a series of toxic effects are produced. Various organs and functions of the body are influenced, and the results of the poison may be briefly summed up as follows:—The intellectual faculties are blunted, the memory is impaired, the ideas confused, the patient is dull, stupid, and apathetic, and has a constant tendency to somnolence. The speech is impeded and slow, and the tongue is tremulous. The special senses are weakened. The body, as a whole, is infirm, the limbs feeble, and the gait staggering and incoördinated. The reflex excitability is lowered and the sensibility diminished. The sexual

powers are impaired or abolished. These symptoms may be present in a variety of degrees, and in advanced cases even imbecility or paralysis may ensue. The mucous membranes become dry and insensitive, especially those of the fauces. This is attended with various functional disorders, such as nausea, flatulence, gastric catarrh, diarrhœa, &c. The skin is pale, and the extremities are cold. The action of the heart is slow and weak. The respiration is shallow, hurried, and imperfect. The integument is frequently covered with an acne-like eruption. To these symptoms may be added a general cachexia. All these abnormal conditions, as a rule, disappear when the consumption of the poison is arrested.

2. Although some persons, suffering from epileptic seizures, are, in the intervals, of sound mind and body, in many the inter-paroxysmal state is characterized by certain symptoms peculiar to this condition, and independent of any form of treatment. These vary from the slightest departures from health to the most serious mental and physical disease. The general health is frequently unsatisfactory; the functions of the body being impaired in vigour, the digestion is weak, and the circulation feeble. The entire nervous system is in an unstable condition, the patient being at one time irritable and excitable, and at another depressed and despondent. There is a very common condition of so-called "nervousness" which is accompanied by headache, pains, tremors, and a variety of other subjective phenomena. The mental powers are enfeebled, the memory defective, and these intellectual alterations may exist in any degree, even to permanent and intractable forms of insanity. The physical conditions may also be changed, the nutrition of the tissues is often imperfect, the skin is pale, the muscles flabby, and the motor powers generally enfeebled, all of which may also present different degrees of severity, so as to culminate in actual paralysis.

Admitting, then, that the prolonged and excessive administration of the bromides causes a series of abnormal symptoms in the healthy individual, affecting mainly the general nutrition, the mental faculties, and the sensory and motor functions, and also that the epileptic state is itself frequently accompanied by impairment of innervation of a somewhat analogous nature, it follows that when the drug is given for the relief of the disease, care must be taken not to confound the two series of phenomena with one another. With this precaution in view, granting that the therapeutic agent beneficially controls and suppresses the convulsive seizures, we proceed to discuss whether in so doing it in any way injuriously influences the constitution of the patient. To answer this question has been found by no means easy. Comparatively few physicians have opportunities of observing cases of epilepsy in sufficient numbers to form substantial conclusions on the subject. Even in favoured circumstances it is difficult, especially in hospital practice, to ensure the regular attendance of the patient or to keep him sufficiently long under observation. The study and the recording of the facts, moreover, demand an expenditure of much time and labour. These, added to the sources of fallacy already enumerated, render the inquiry a complicated one; but it is believed that an approximation to the truth may be arrived at by the following method of investigation.

A large number of cases of epilepsy form the basis of the statistics, the great majority of whom are adults. No selection of any kind is made, and all are admitted irrespective of the cause, nature, or severity of the disease. The particulars of each having been noted, treatment by the bromides was instituted, the minimum dose being one drachm and a half daily,[G] which, if necessary, was further increased in quantity. The progress of the patient was observed at frequent and regular intervals, and if the attendance was irregular the case was excluded from the present inquiry. The result of this proceeding is an aggregate of 141 cases, all of whom have been constantly under the influence of the drug for periods varying from one to six years. These are arranged in groups according to the length of time they were under treatment. The immense mass of details thus collected, added to the varied circumstances connected with individual cases, render it impossible, in constructing a summary of the whole, to do more than select certain prominent features of interest for examination and demonstration. These in tabular form are as follows:—

TABLES SHOWING THE EFFECTS OF THE CONTINUOUS ADMINISTRATION OF THE BROMIDES IN THE EPILEPTIC STATE, IN 141 CASES, THE CONDITION BEING ASCERTAINED AT THE END OF EACH PERIOD.

I. *For one year (51 cases).*

Physical and mental powers unaffected	39, or 76.4 per cent.
Physical and mental powers impaired	6, or 11.7 per cent.
Physical powers alone impaired	3, or 5.9 per cent.
Mental powers alone impaired	2, or 3.9 per cent.
General symptoms of neurasthenia	13, or 25.4 per cent.
Bromide eruption	8, or 15.6 per cent.

II. *For two years (34 cases).*

Physical and mental powers unaffected	28, or 82.3 per cent.
Physical and mental powers impaired	2, or 5.8 per cent.
Physical powers alone impaired	1, or 2.9 per cent.

Mental powers alone impaired	2, or 5.8 per cent.
General symptoms of neurasthenia	5, or 14.7 per cent.
Bromide eruption	6, or 17.6 per cent.

III. *For three years (30 cases).*

Physical and mental powers unaffected	28, or 93.3 per cent.
Physical and mental powers impaired	1, or 3.3 per cent.
Physical powers alone impaired	1, or 3.3 per cent.
Mental powers alone impaired	0, or 0.0 per cent.
General symptoms of neurasthenia	3, or 10.0 per cent.
Bromide eruption	3, or 10.0 per cent.

IV. *For four years (16 cases).*

Physical and mental powers unaffected	12, or 75.0 per cent.
Physical and mental powers impaired	0, or 0.0 per cent.
Physical powers alone impaired	2, or 12.5 per cent.
Mental powers alone impaired	2, or 12.5 per cent.
General symptoms of neurasthenia	0, or 0.0 per cent.
Bromide eruption	2, or 12.5 per cent.

V. *For five years (6 cases).*

Physical and mental powers unaffected	6, or 100.0 per cent.
Physical and mental powers impaired	0, or 0.0 per cent.
Physical powers alone impaired	0, or 0.0 per cent.
Mental powers alone impaired	0, or 0.0 per cent.
General symptoms of neurasthenia	3, or 50.0 per cent.
Bromide eruption	0, or 0.0 per cent.

VI. *For six years (4 cases).*

Physical and mental powers unaffected	4, or 100.0 per cent.
Physical and mental powers impaired	0, or 0.0 per cent.

Physical powers alone impaired	0, or 0.0 per cent.
Mental powers alone impaired	0, or 0.0 per cent.
General symptoms of neurasthenia	2, or 50.0 per cent.
Bromide eruption	0, or 0.0 per cent.

In the construction of the details of the above tables, care has been taken as far as possible to distinguish between the effects of the remedy and the symptoms associated with the disease, although this has not been always easy to accomplish. It has, however, been approximately arrived at by a careful study of the patient's health before treatment, as compared with his subsequent state, and those symptoms only were considered toxic which were superadded to pre-existing abnormal conditions. A general analysis of the facts thus collected shows that in the majority of cases the physical and mental powers do not appear to be injuriously affected by the prolonged use of the bromides. It is not asserted that all the individuals placed under this section were necessarily sound in mind and body. In many instances the functions of these were impaired, but there was no evidence to indicate that this was the result of the medicine taken; on the contrary, there was every reason to believe that the symptoms thus displayed were a part of the original disease, and had existed prior to treatment.

In a very small percentage of cases were both physical and mental powers unfavourably modified as a direct consequence of the use of the bromides, and even in these there is no absolute certainty that the drugs were entirely responsible for the symptoms, seeing that these might be attributed to the epileptic condition as well as to the toxic effects of the remedy. They are considered under this category, as the abnormal phenomena appeared to be augmented after treatment and improved on its temporary cessation. They mainly consisted, on the one hand, of loss of memory, dulness of apprehension, apathy, somnolence, depression of spirits, and mental debility; and on the other, of bodily languor, muscular fatigue, and general physical weakness. In no case did any of these symptoms attain an excessive or prominent position. The same conditions apply when the physical or mental powers were impaired independently of one another.

Under the heading of general phenomena of neurasthenia is included a series of indefinite subjective neurotic symptoms, without intellectual or bodily deficiencies, in which the patient complained of headache, neuralgic pains, tremors, of being easily startled and frightened, with that general instability of the nervous system to which the term neurasthenia has been given. This condition is extremely common in the epileptic, and is frequently relieved by treatment. At other times it remains persistent in spite of all medicaments, and the numbers in the tables indicate those cases conspicuous by their continuance under the use of the bromides. Those attacked by the follicular rash are seen at first to be about 16 per cent., but gradually diminishing in number as the treatment becomes chronic, and finally disappearing altogether.

In addition to the points referred to in the tables, other questions have been investigated, although on a smaller scale. For example, in persons who have been under the influence of the bromides for many years, the skin and tendon reflex action remain intact, and I have never seen a case in which the knee-jerk or plantar phenomena were absent. In only one case was the general sensibility of the skin perceptibly diminished. With regard to the effects on the sexual powers, I have not sufficient data upon which to found positive rules. This statement, however, may be made, that the prolonged use of even large doses of this drug does not of necessity abolish or even sensibly impair this function, although, no doubt, it usually does so. On examining the respiration and pulse, I have never been able to detect any characteristic abnormality.

I might record many cases in detail to prove the seemingly innocuous nature of even large and long-continued doses of the bromides in epilepsy. I shall, however, as an illustration, limit myself to a few notes on the four cases which compose Table VI., all of whom were continuously under the influence of the drugs for a period of not less than six years.

CASE 1.—Louisa C——, aged twenty-nine, has suffered from epileptic attacks for fourteen years. Prior to treatment she had three or four every week, of a severe character, consisting of loss of consciousness, general convulsions, biting of the tongue, &c. She has always been a delicate person, with a tendency to great nervousness, but otherwise intelligent, and in fair general health. She has taken one and a half drachms of bromide of potassium daily regularly for the last six years, and states that if she attempts to discontinue the medicine all her symptoms are aggravated. At present the patient is a robust, healthy-looking woman, of fair intelligence and good spirits. Her memory is deficient. Her physical powers are vigorous, and she earns her living as a bookbinder. She has an attack about once a month, and with the exception of this and occasional headaches and nervousness, she professes and seems to be in excellent general health. Sensibility, the knee-jerk, and plantar phenomena are normal. The fauces are insensitive, and their reflex is abolished. Pulse 60, normal. The circulation, respiration, and other functions are healthy. No traces of bromism.

CASE 2.—Charles P——, aged thirty-five, has suffered from epileptic attacks of a severe convulsive character for eighteen years, having had one about once a month. Prior to treatment, although his memory was defective, his intelligence and general health were good. For the last six years he has regularly taken the bromides of potassium and ammonium (one drachm and a half) daily. At present he still continues to have an attack about once a month. His mental and physical conditions are the same as before. He appears perfectly intelligent. His strength is robust, so that he does his ordinary work as a pianoforte maker. Pulse 74, of good strength. All the reflexes are normal, except that of the fauces, which is abolished. Sensibility of the skin to touch slightly diminished. The sexual functions are normal. No symptoms of bromism.

CASE 3.—Matilda W——, aged thirty-one, has suffered from epilepsia gravior and mitior for twenty-two years, having of the former about one seizure in three months, and of the latter ten or twelve a day. She has always been a delicate woman, suffering from headaches, general irritability, and nervousness. She is, however, perfectly intelligent. For six years past she has taken regularly the bromides of potassium and ammonium, one drachm of each daily. She has not had an attack of epilepsy major for a year, and of epilepsy mitior has now only about one a week. Although anæmic, her general health is good, and she is able to do a full day's work as a washer-woman. Intellectually she is quite sound, but has a treacherous memory, and is very nervous. Sensibility, reflex acts, &c., are as in the other cases.

CASE 4.—Lucy D——, aged twenty-two, has suffered from epilepsy major for eight years. Formerly had about one attack a week. Has always been a delicate girl, but her general health and mental condition have been normal. For the last six years she has regularly taken one drachm and a half of the bromides daily (potassium and ammonium in equal parts). She has had only three attacks during the past year. Her general health is excellent. She is robust and active, and takes her full share in domestic work. She is well educated, intelligent, with good memory and spirits, and has no tendency to depression or somnolence. The sensibility, reflex acts, and other functions are as in the other cases.

In these four cases it has been ascertained that the patients were constantly under the influence of large doses of the bromides for a period of not less than six years, and practically without intermission. During this period not only were the frequency and severity of the convulsive attacks beneficially modified, but there was no evidence to show that the physical or mental condition had been in any way impaired. It is further to be observed that these as well as many others of those constituting the later tables, are examples of unusually long-standing and severe forms of epilepsy, as evidenced by the fact of their chronic and intractable nature even under treatment. Notwithstanding the incompleteness of their recovery, these individuals have voluntarily, and often at great inconvenience and expense, persevered in the use of the remedy, which is a fair indication they derived some substantial benefit from it. The examples before us, one and all, declared they have found by experience that when they have attempted, even for brief periods, to discontinue the medicine their symptoms have all become aggravated. As a result the attacks increase in severity and number, the headaches return, the nervousness augments, and they are unable to perform either mental or bodily exertion. These sufferings, it is maintained, are greatly modified by the bromides, as under their influence epileptics may perform their daily work, when without them they are comparatively useless. It would be easy to multiply individual cases supporting the same general principles. One more instance only need be particularized—namely, that of a man aged thirty, who has suffered from epilepsy from infancy, and who for the last five years has taken *four and a half drachms* of the bromides daily—*i.e.*, during that time he has consumed upwards of *eighty pounds* of the drug. Although a delicate person and intellectually weak, his friends state that during those years he has been more healthy and robust in mind and body than at any other period of his life. And these statements were confirmed by other testimony.

While attempting to estimate the therapeutic value of the bromides from a statistical aspect, one likely source of fallacy must not be overlooked. Most patients, and especially those attending hospitals, are difficult to keep under observation for long periods, more particularly if the progress of the case is unsatisfactory. In this way we may lose sight of those who do not benefit by treatment or who are injured by it. Although it is difficult to estimate these with accuracy, a certain rebatement must always be made on this count in computing results. At the same time we have in the present inquiry positive evidence, in a considerable number of cases, of the innocuous and beneficial nature of the drug, against the negative possibility only of its disadvantages. Of the 141 cases under notice, I only know of three who have died, and all of then of phthisis pulmonalis. The relations existing between the mortality and cause of death on the one hand, and the disease and treatment on the other, the paucity of the data do not permit us to determine.

A further study of the tables would also seem to show that while the beneficial action of the bromides remains permanent, the deleterious effects diminish the longer the drug has been taken. This is doubtless due, as in the case of most poisons, to the system becoming habituated to its use. It has often been observed that the most marked effects of bromism have appeared at the beginning of treatment, and that the eruption, the physical and mental depression, &c., subsequently disappeared, although the medicine was persevered in. Those who have been under its influence for some years rarely present any symptoms directly attributable to the toxic effects of the bromides; and if abnormal conditions do exist, these are the sequelæ of the malady, and not the results of treatment, as shown by the fact that when the last is suspended, the original sufferings are augmented.

It may be suggested that a prolonged use of the bromides becomes, as in the case of opium, a habit. There is, however, a marked distinction between the two. Opium-smoking is a vice not only deleterious in itself, but one indulged in merely to satisfy a morbid craving. The bromides, on the other hand, are less hurtful in their effects, and are taken to avert the symptoms of a distressing and terrible malady. Assuming, then, that their consumption becomes a necessity, if it can be shown that the results are not serious, while the evils they avert are important, the habit acquired may be looked upon as a justifiable one.

A general review of all these circumstances seems to render it probable that the epileptic constitution is more tolerant of the toxic effects of the bromides than the healthy system. The most severe effects of bromism occur in those who are not the victims of this malady, in whom, as seen by the foregoing facts, they are not common. Theoretically this may be plausibly explained by the reasonable assumption that, as in epilepsy the entire nervous apparatus is in a state of reflex hyper-excitability, the sedative and poisonous effects of the bromides do not produce the depressing or toxic actions they would do in a more stable organization. Whatever the reason may be, the fact is that the symptoms of bromism are not so severe in the epileptic as they are in otherwise healthy subjects.

Finally, the important question arises, Does a prolonged use of the bromides tend towards the eradication of the disease itself and the ultimate cure of the epileptic state? On this point I have no personal statistical evidence to offer, nor am I aware of the existence of any sufficiently scientific series of data to settle the question. Without there being actual demonstration of the fact, there is every reason to believe that such a supposition is possible. Clinical observation has determined that the larger the number of convulsive seizures the greater is the tendency to the production of others, and the more readily are they caused. Such is the abnormal reflex hyper-excitability of the nervous system of the epileptic that the irritative effects of one attack seem directly to pre-dispose to the occurrence of a second; so that the larger the number of explosions of nerve instability which actually take place, the more there are likely to follow. Could such seizures be kept in check, this cause of the production of convulsions at least would be diminished, the liability for them to break out as a result of trifling external stimuli would be lessened, and the long-continued absence of this source of irritation might by the repose and favourable circumstances thus obtained, encourage a healthy transformation of tissue. Now, it has already been pointed out that in 12.1 per cent. of epileptics the attacks were completely arrested during the entire time the drugs were being administered, and that in a much larger percentage they were greatly modified in number and severity. It has been further shown that the remedies themselves, even when in use for long periods, are in themselves practically innocuous, while at the same time they continue to maintain their beneficial effects on the attacks. It therefore follows that a sufficiently prolonged treatment might in a certain number of cases be succeeded by permanent curative results. The chief impediment to arriving at trustworthy conclusions on this subject has been the length of time necessary to judge of lasting benefits, and the difficulty of keeping patients sufficiently long under observation. Another has been the objection raised to the method of treatment on the grounds of a visionary suspicion that the toxic effects of the drug were of a dangerous nature, and their results more distressing than the diseases for which they were given. So far as my experience has extended, I believe this fear has not been warranted by facts.

FOOTNOTES:

[D] Reprinted from the "Lancet" of May 17th and 24th, 1884.

[E] See Article II.

[F] Vide preceding paper.

[G] The usual prescription contained the bromides of potassium and ammonium, fifteen grains of each for a dose.

June, 1884.

Milton Keynes UK
Ingram Content Group UK Ltd.
UKHW030002260824
447288UK00004B/211